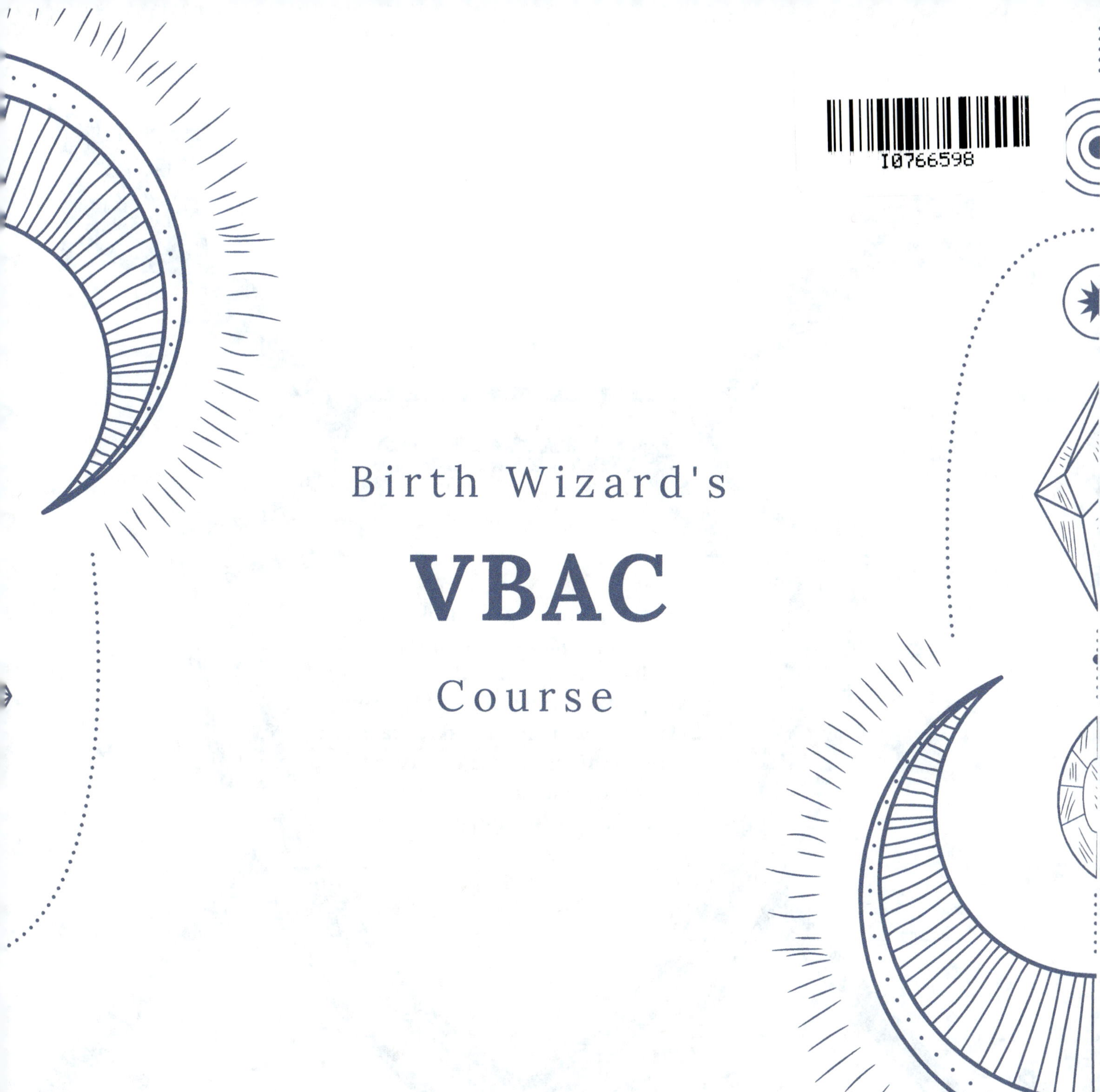

Birth Wizard's

VBAC

Course

School of the Birth Wizardry
Tome of Birth Wisdom
Volume I: VBAC

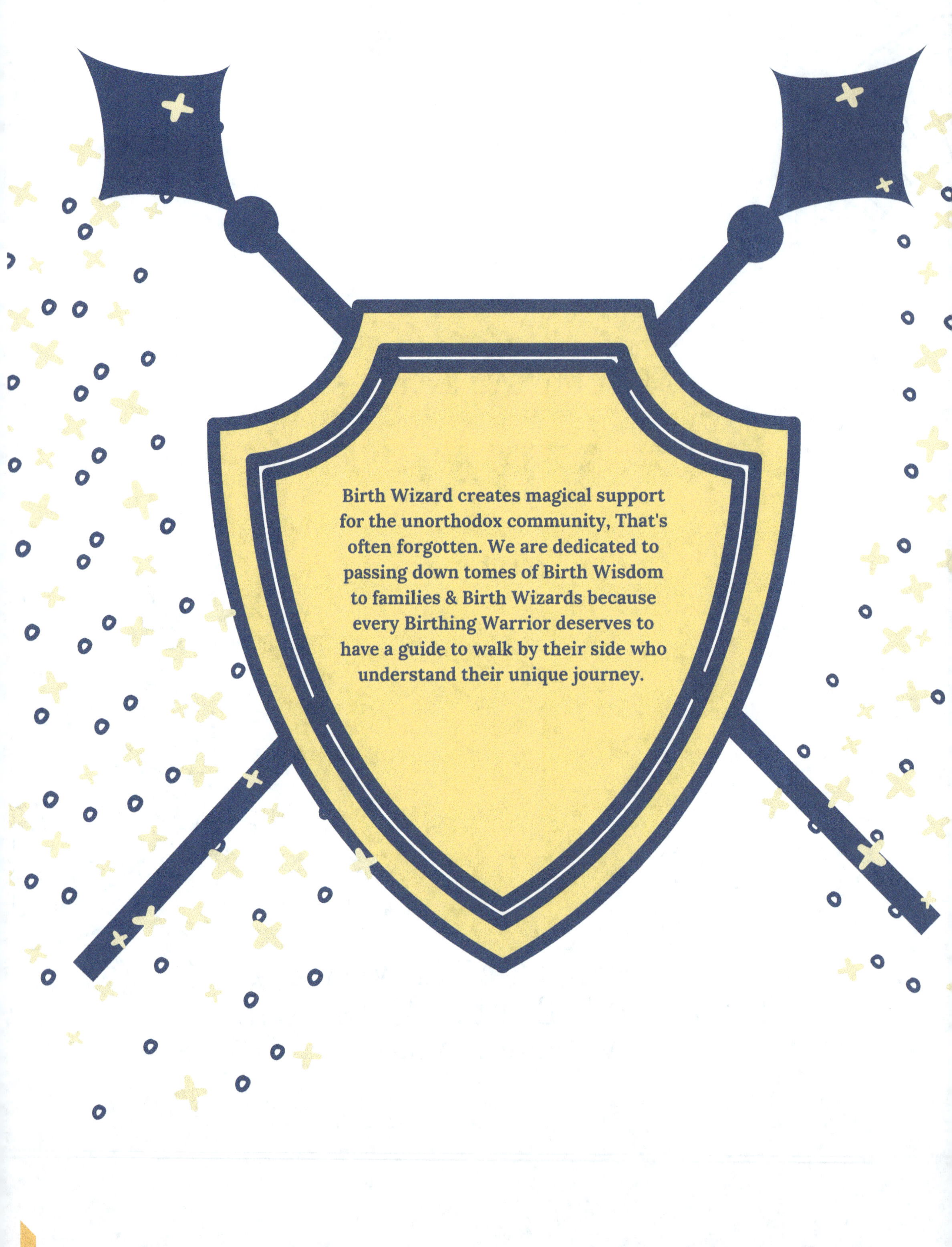

Birth Wizard creates magical support for the unorthodox community, That's often forgotten. We are dedicated to passing down tomes of Birth Wisdom to families & Birth Wizards because every Birthing Warrior deserves to have a guide to walk by their side who understand their unique journey.

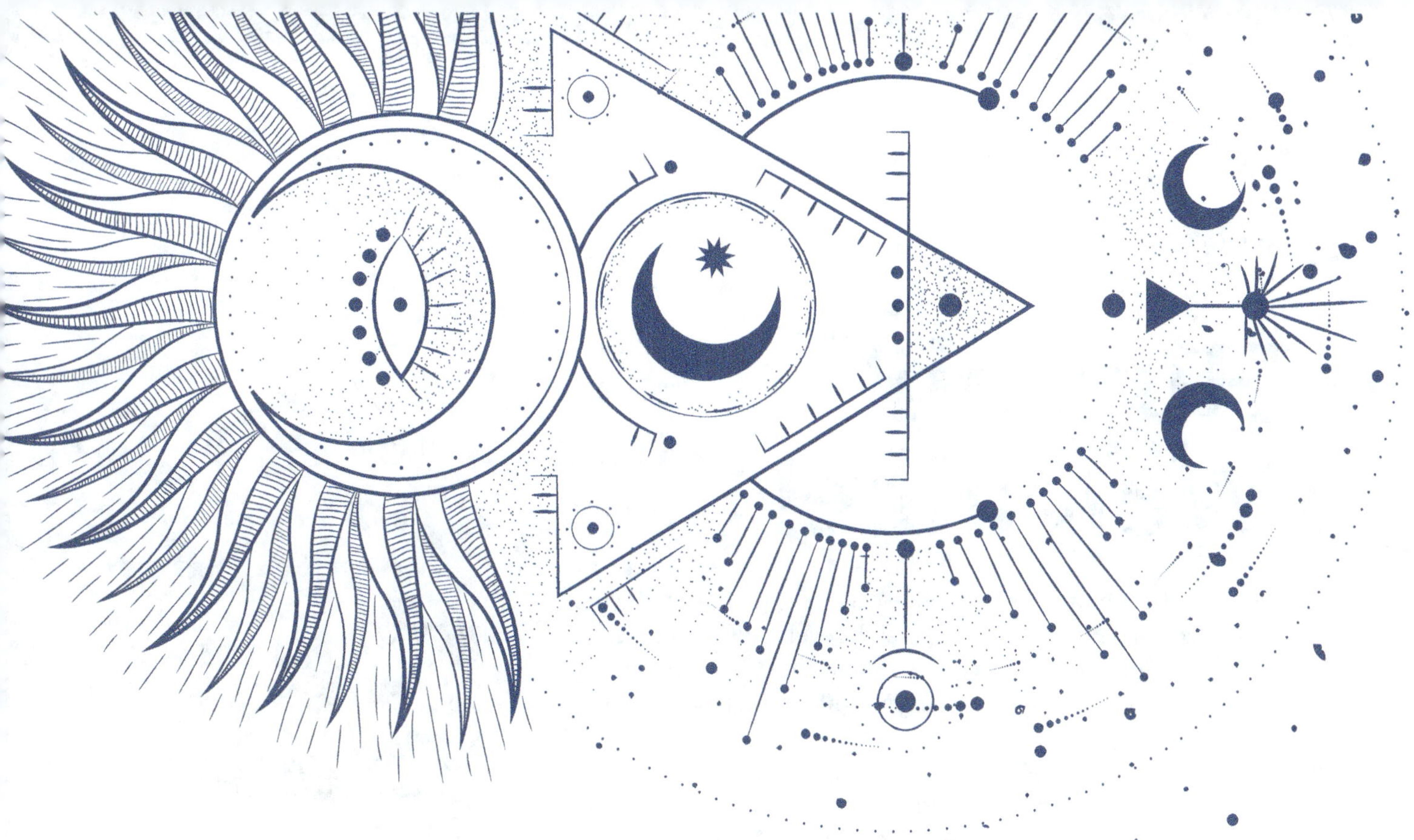

Table of Contents

Huzzah! Welcome!

I appreciate you taking this unique class to guide through your VBAC journey. This class was developed with care, understanding and knowing how important this is to you. My own quest for VBAC is what led me to be an advocate, doula and educator.

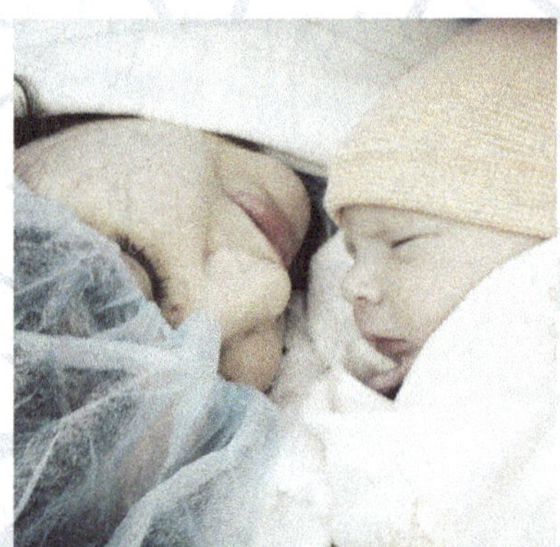

My first pregnancy "was a dream" and assumed that childbirth would be the same. I was the "perfect patient", meaning never questioned anything the doctor's or hospital told me, and like 1 in 3 women in America, this resulted in a c-section. The operative report from c-section references my weight as the reason I couldn't give birth vaginally, which was hurtful and felt wrong. My body couldn't be the problem - I've always been athletic and strong physically, despite any pregnancy weight. It lit a fire in my heart to figure out how it all happened, with the intent of making my next birth a VBAC.

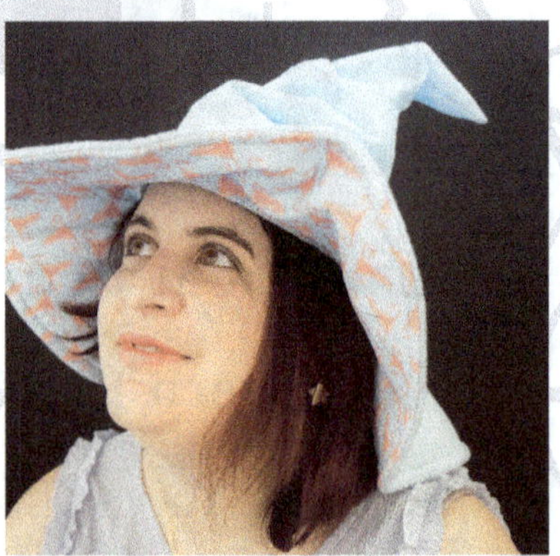

I spent almost a year researching, joining groups, attending therapy, and reading everything I could get my hands on about vaginal birth and c-sections. All that work paid off and I've gone on to have TWO successful VBAC births, and most importantly - healed my birth trauma.

Your Birth Wizard is always excited to help with any extra assistance you need on your journey. I'm always excited to hear from participants of this course. Summon any Birth Wizard by sending an email or carrier pigeon.

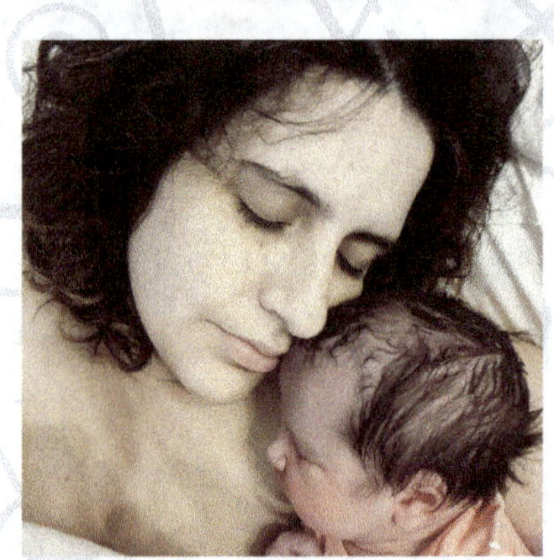

Here's to you and your future empowered birth

Emmy Howard

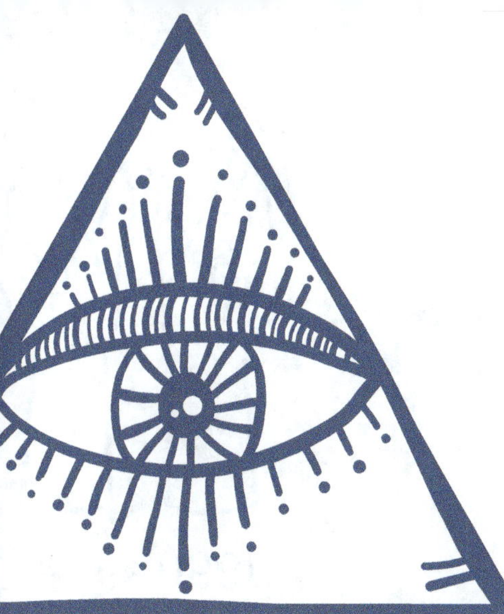

Ancient History

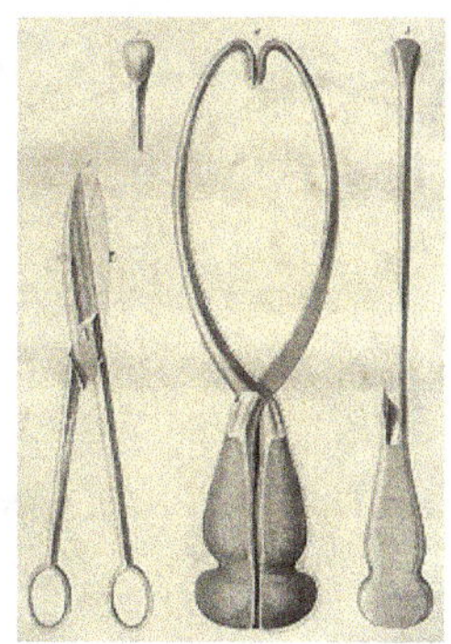

_____________ clan in England introduced obstetrical forceps to pull from the birth canal fetuses in _____'s

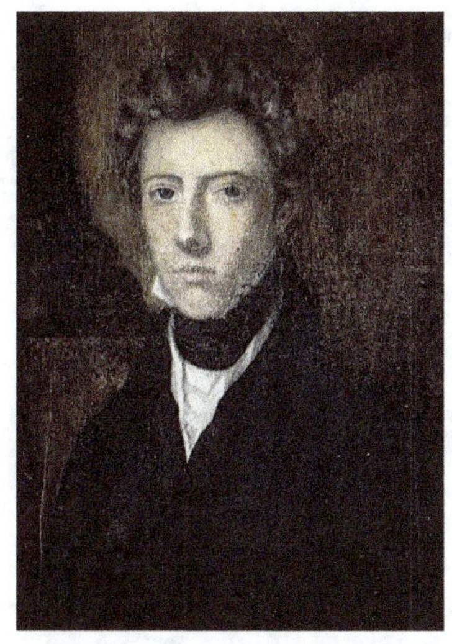

______ ______ is famous for performing first successful cesarean birth in United Kingdom

Skills he picked up from the indigenous people of ______ Kingdom

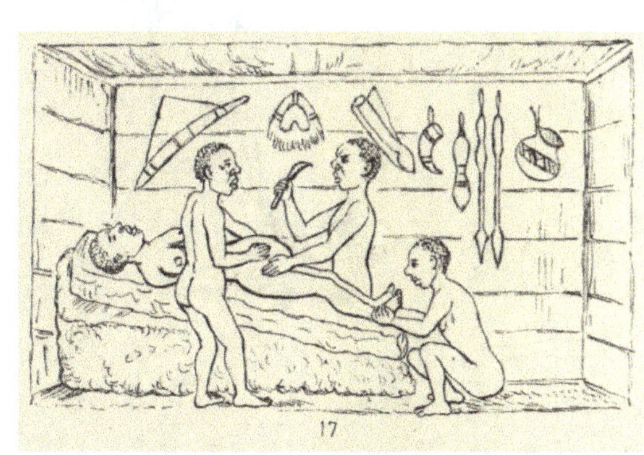

Modern History

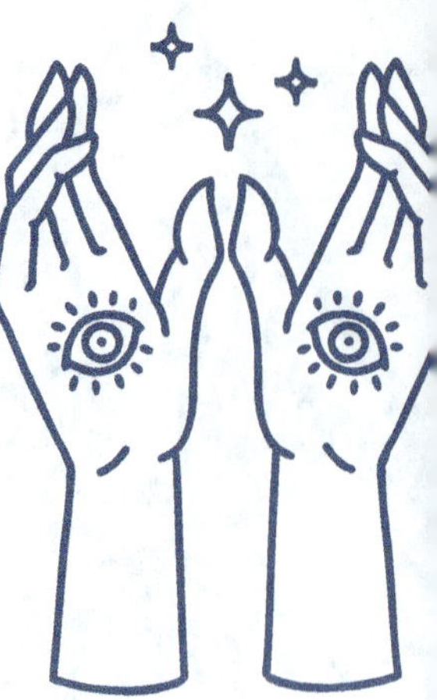

1970's

1980's

1990's

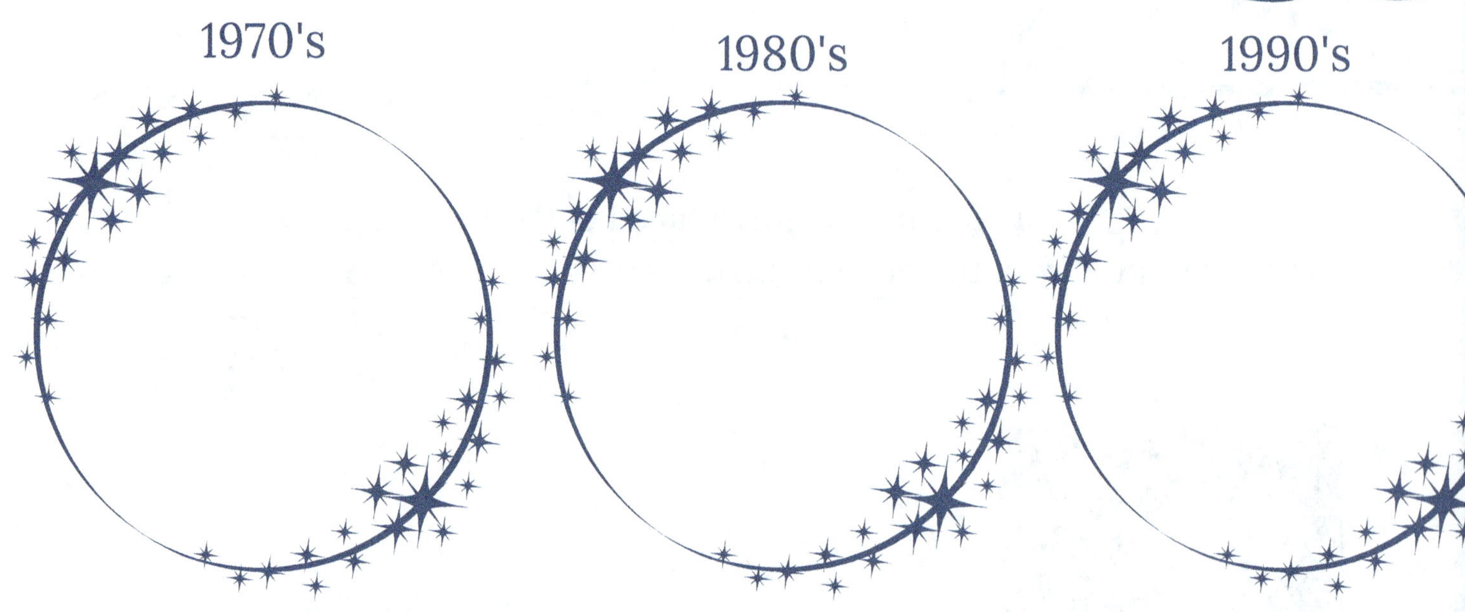

In 2018 ~__% was the national Cesarean Rate

2006

2010

2016

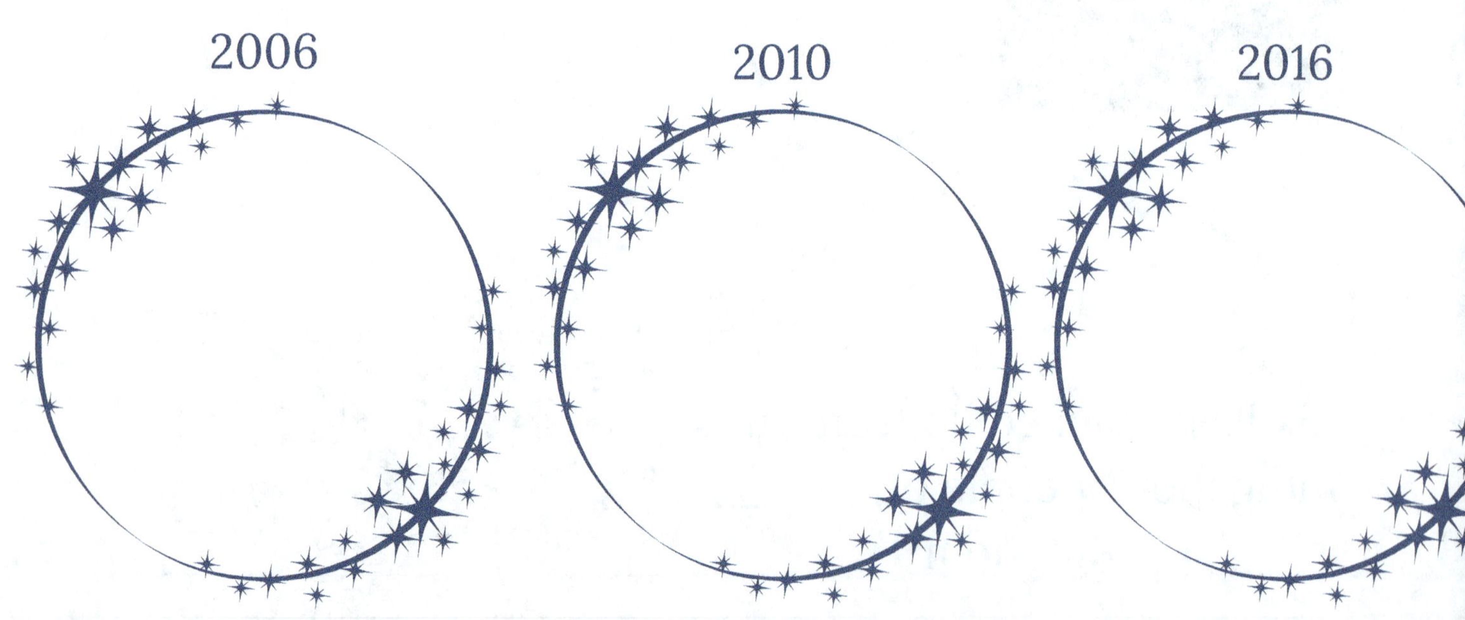

Obstacles:VBAC

Fill in the States VBAC Laws Covered

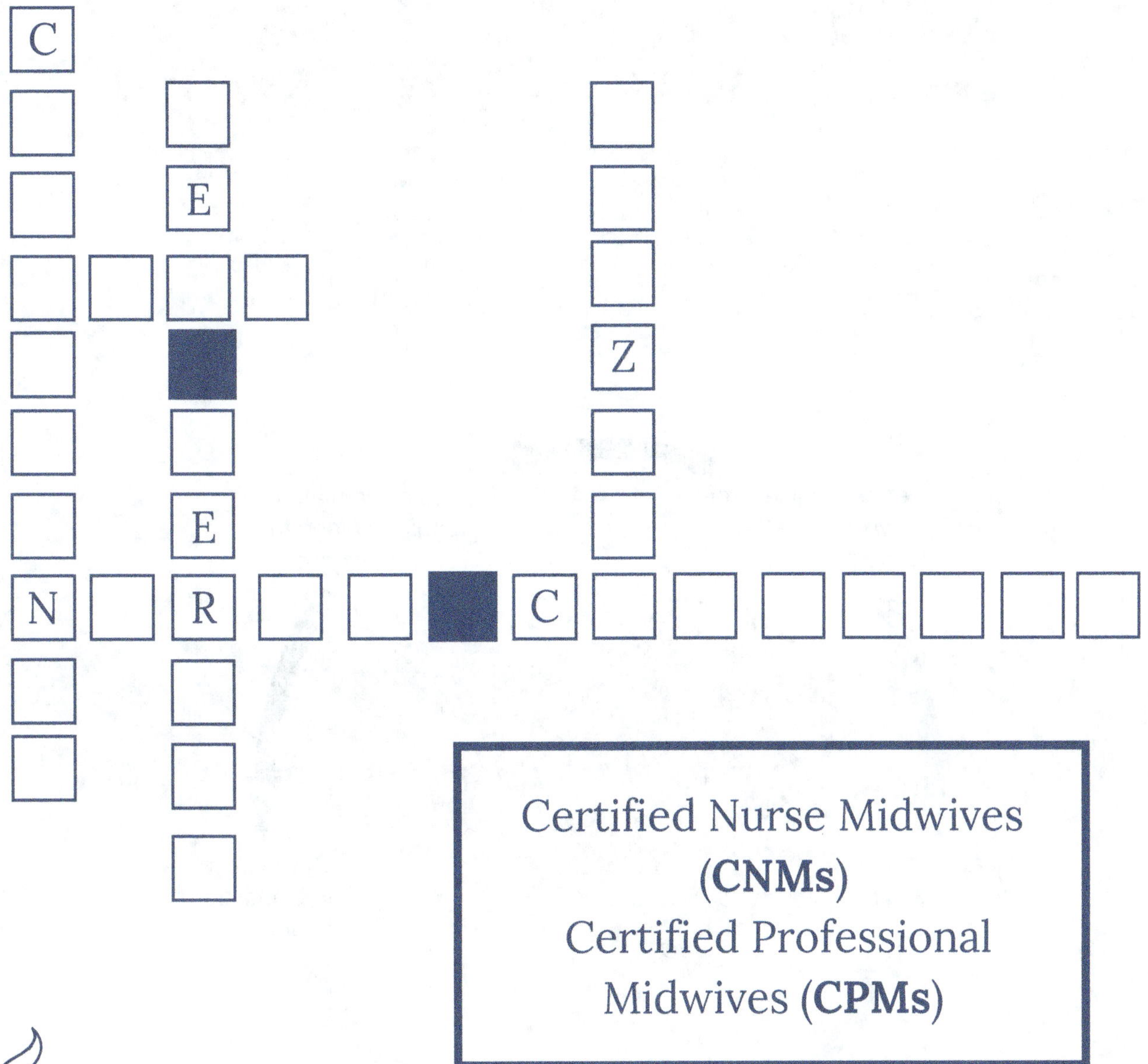

Certified Nurse Midwives **(CNMs)**
Certified Professional Midwives **(CPMs)**

Body, Brain & Baby

Cervical Effacement

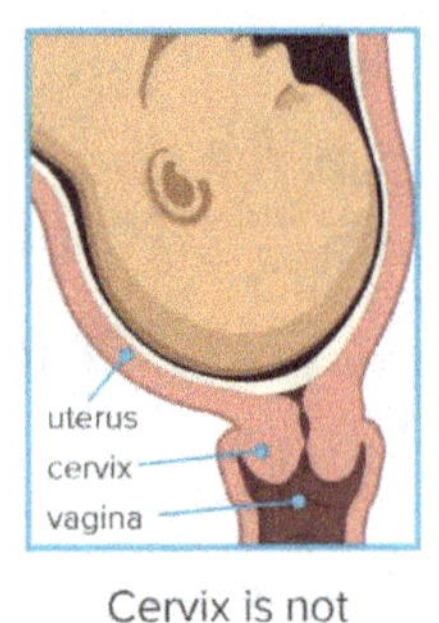

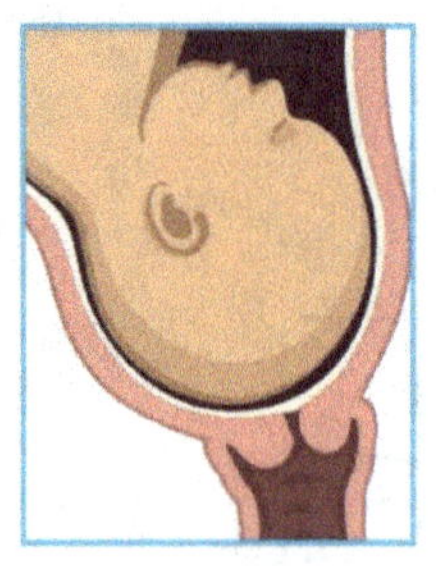

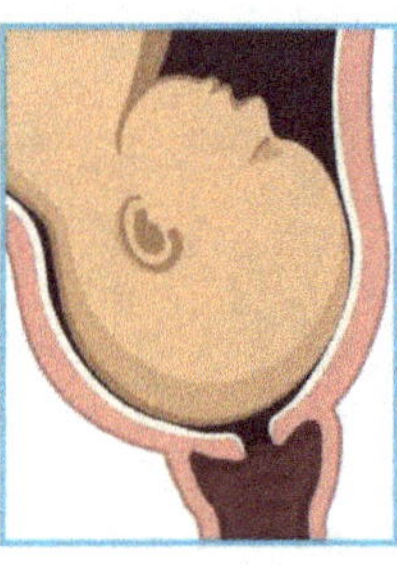

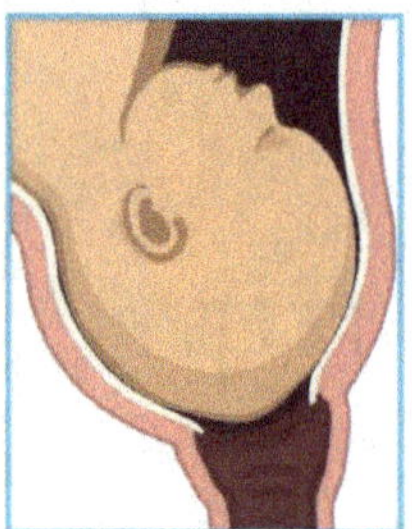

Cervix is not effaced or dilated

Cervix is 50% effaced and not dilated

Cervix is 100% effaced and dilated to 3 cm

Cervix is fully dilated to 10 cm

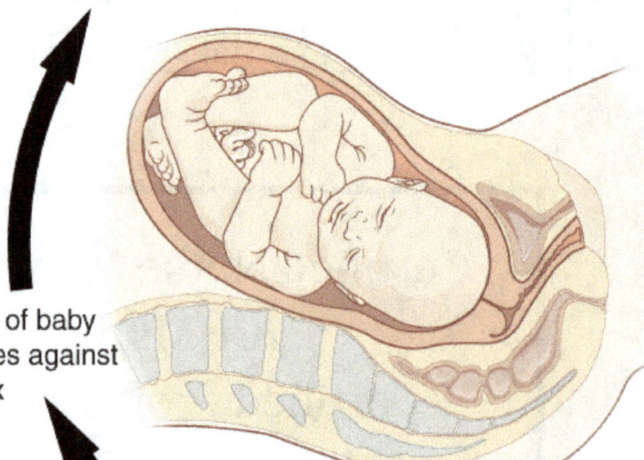

Magic of Labor

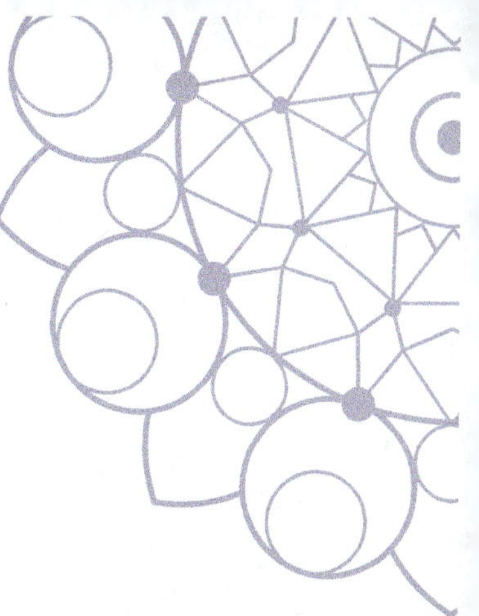

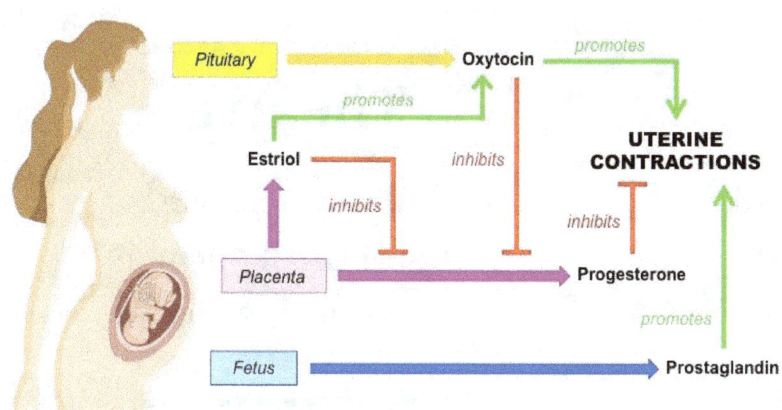

Brain Chemistry

Oxytocin
Endorphins
Catecholamines
Prolactin

Brain Waves

Beta

Alpha

Theta

Delta

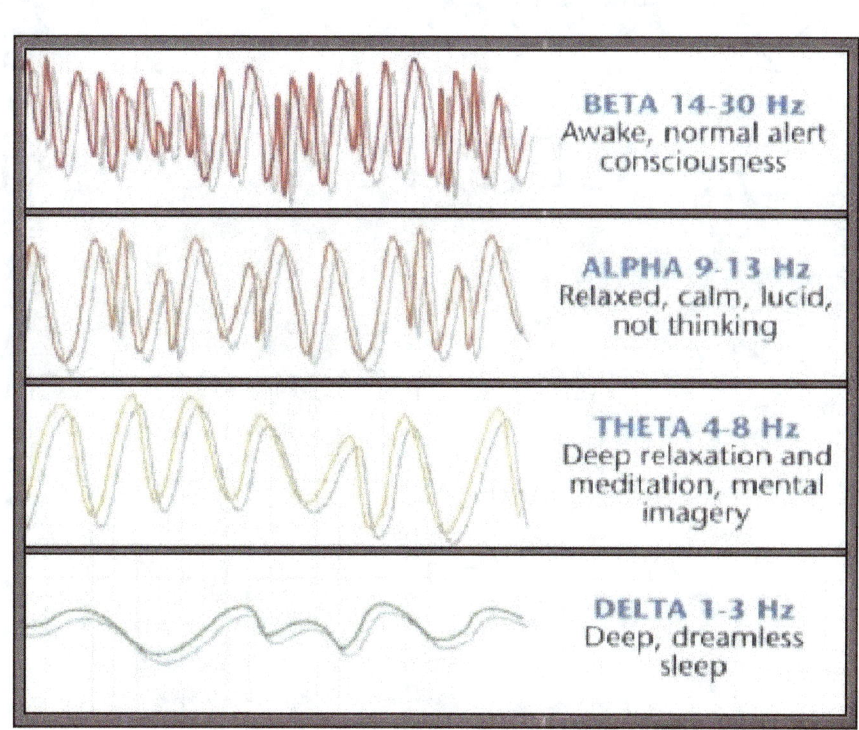

Dilation

the action or condition of becoming or being made wider, larger, or more open.

0-10 cm

Concert

Curtains are open but show isn't ready to start

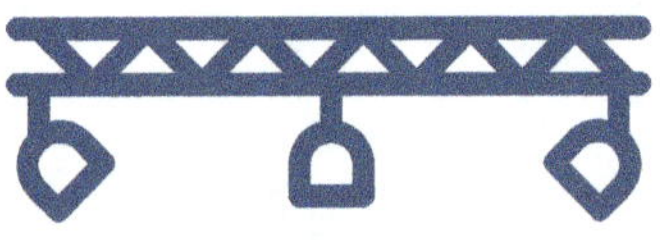

Theatre

Curtains stayed closed until show is ready to start

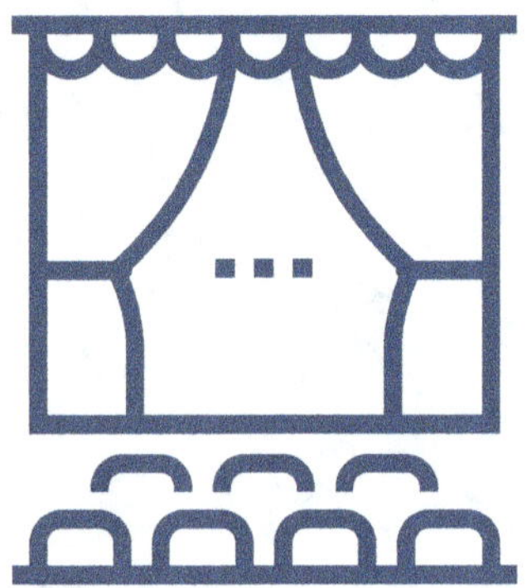

CERVICAL DILATION

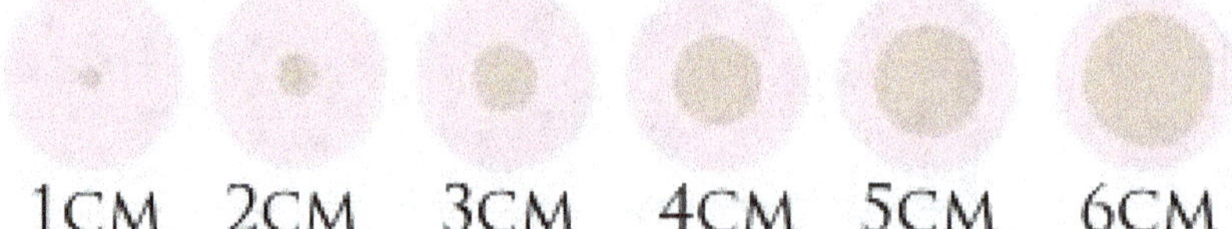

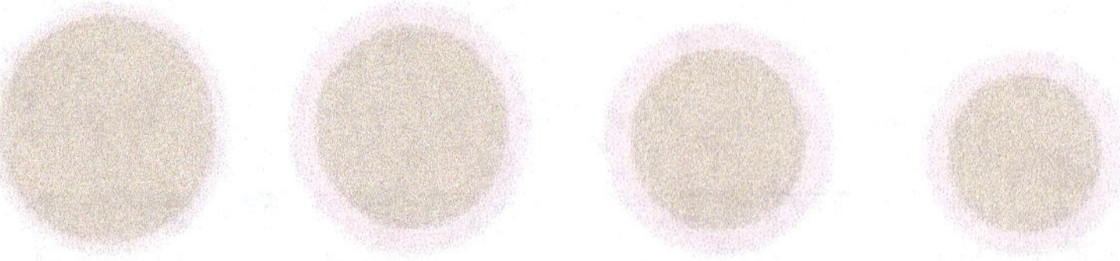

THIS CERVICAL DILATION CHART IS AN APPROXIMATE MEASURE OF CERVICAL DILATION.

STATION

the baby's presenting part–most likely the head–
in relation to the ischial spines of the birther's
pelvis

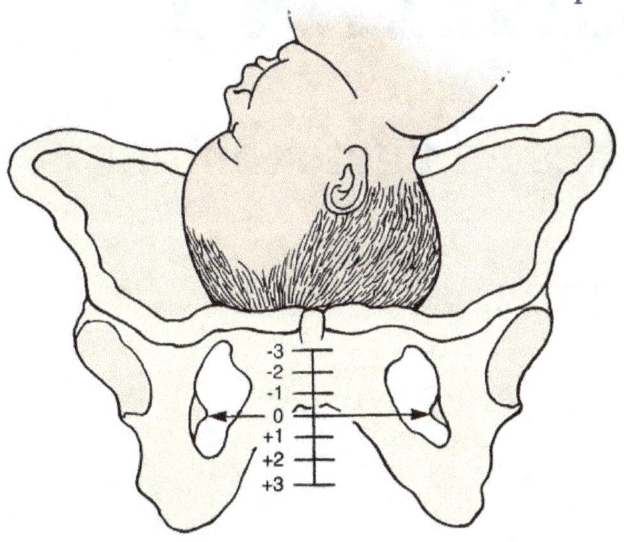

Understood on a number line
-4 to +4

Just like a train has stops at the
stations

Most major stop is 0

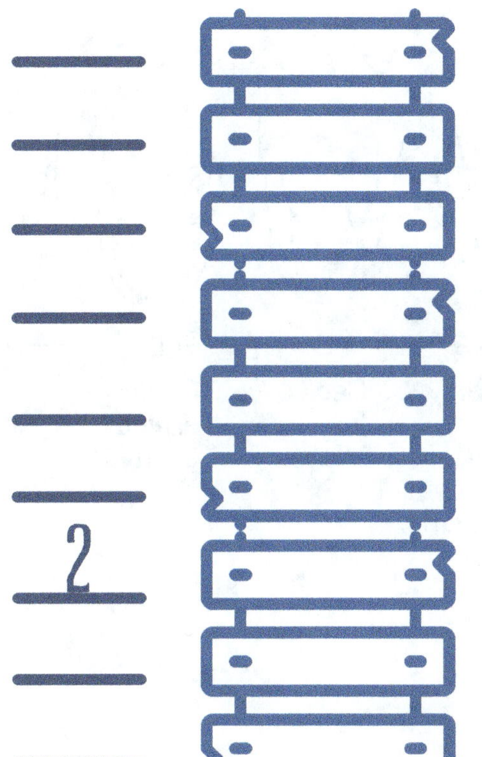
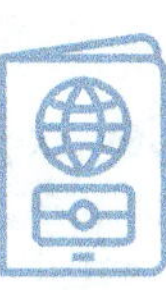

EFFACEMENT

that the cervix stretches and gets thinner

0% to 100%

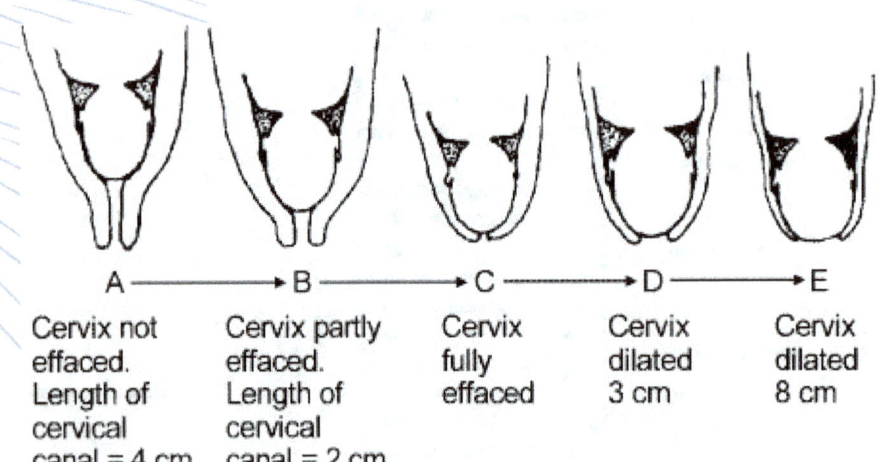

Positioning

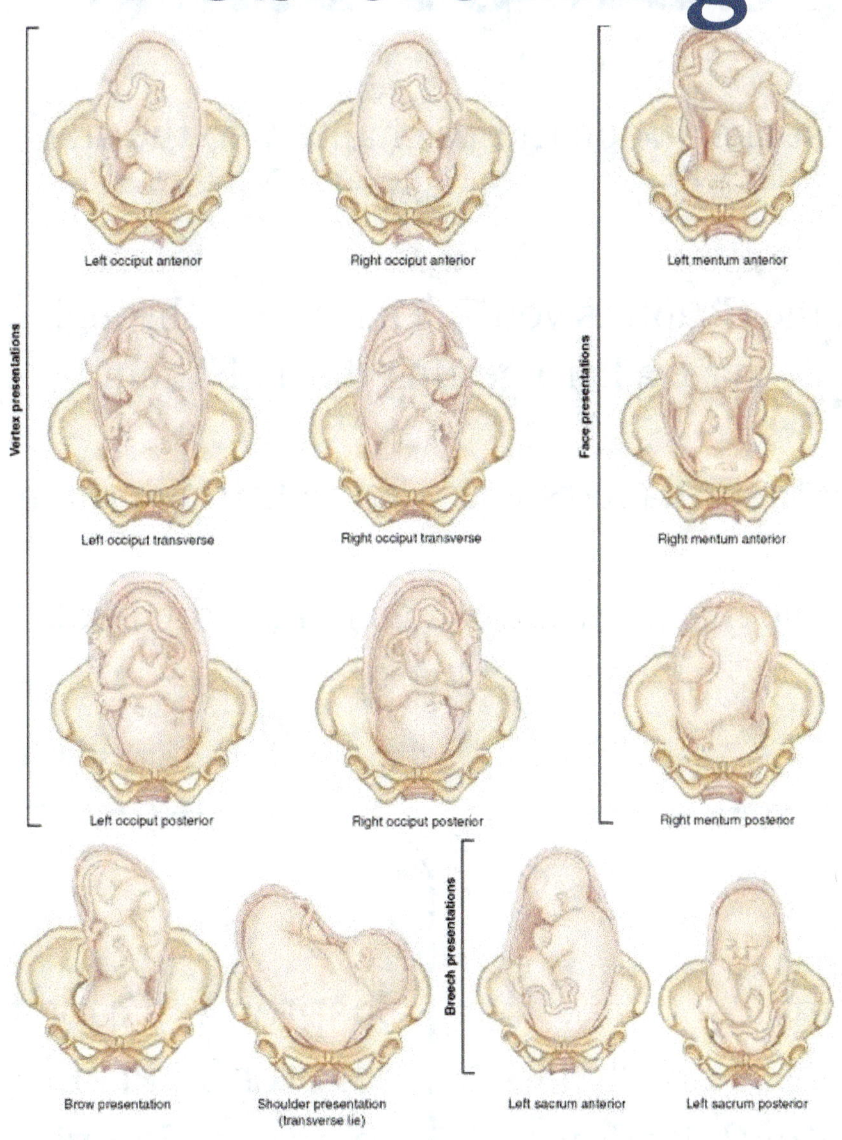

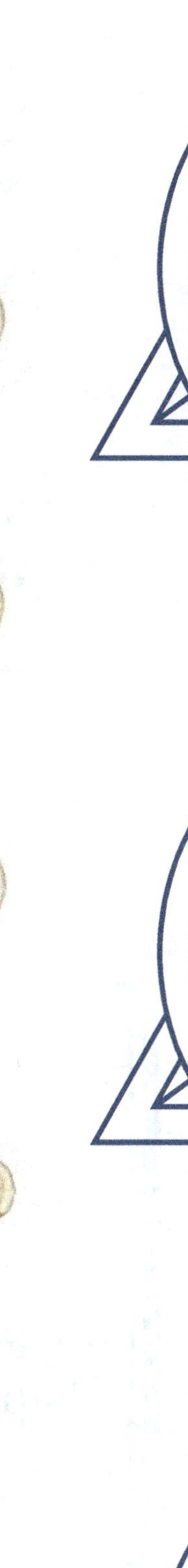

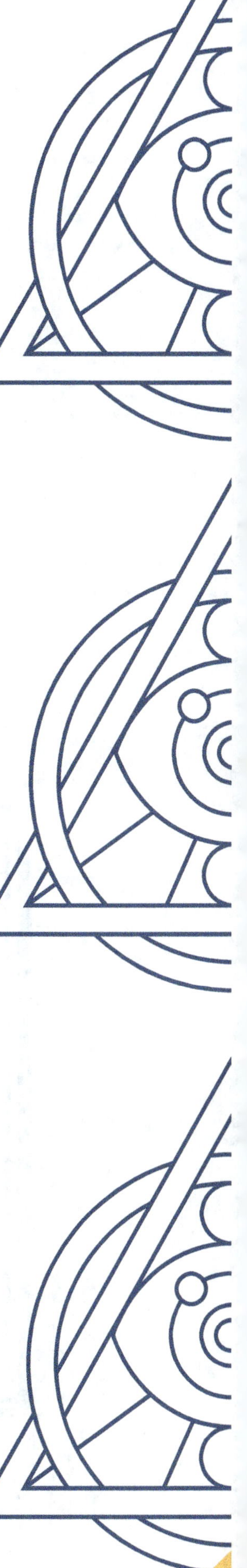

LOA ________________________

ROA ________________________

LOP ________________________

ROP ________________________

BOOK OF LABOR

Just like a book theres chapters to the stages
of labor

Some Chapters you will fall asleep through or
have a hard getting through them

Other Chapters you will wiz through them

No matter what you will finish the book

Preamble

Chapter 1- Early labor

Chapter 2-Bridging

Chapter 3-Active

Chapter 4- Transition

Chapter 5- Pushing

Chapter 6-Baby!

Chapter 7-Placenta

BOOK OF LABOR
Preamble
Circle the ones you have experienced before

Diarrhea

Loose-feeling joints

Fatigue

Lighting Crouch/Quickening

Prodromal Labor

Baby Drops

Weight Gain Stops

Bloody Show

Losing Mucus Plug

Nesting

Water Breaks

Instinct tells you its going to happen

BOOK OF LABOR

Chapter 1: Early Labor

Contractions may have regular pattern and easy to manage

Feelings

Excited

Nervous

Annoyed

Contractions

5-20 mins apart
Not Consistent
Can be ignored

Dilation

0 cm to 4 cm

Effacement

0% to 60%

Things to do

Eat

Sleep

Walk

Go out

Distraction

What will you do as your distractions?

____

____

____

____

BOOK OF LABOR
Chapter 2: Bridging

not clinically in "Active Labor" but you'll feel that way

Feelings

Like you are working
No longer "fun" but not bad
Annoyed
Excited
May Need support

Contractions

5-10 mins apart
Consistent
Managable

Dilation

2 cm to 5 cm

Effacement

20% to 60%

Things to do

Call doula or support

Leaning forward during
contractions may help

Still hanging out in
intial birth space

What are some comfort
measures you have utilized
before?

____

____

____

____

BOOK OF LABOR

Chapter 3: Active

Progress is faster now, more intense

Feelings

Focused
Intensity
Rhythm
Intimidation
Confident

Contractions

2-4 mins apart
Consistent
Intensity picked up

Dilation

3 cm to 8 cm

Effacement

40% to 90%

Things to do

Call doula or support
Stairs
Hip circles
Moaning
Kissing
Dancing
Head to birthing space

What are some items to set up your birthing space personalized?

____

____

____

____

BOOK OF LABOR
Chapter 4: Transition

The last bit of dilation and can be overwhelming

Feelings

Fear
Encouragement
Accomplishment
"Finally"
Powerful/less

Contractions

2-3 mins apart
Consistent
Most Intense

Dilation

7 cm to 9 cm

Effacement

100%

Things to do

Routine
Tub or Shower
Zone Out
Breathe Deeply
Listening to baby/body

What is one way you can tell you are in Transition?

____

____

____

____

BOOK OF LABOR

Chapter 5: Pushing

Complete and feeling pressure

Feelings

Surreal
Tired or Invigorated
Focus
Learning Curve

Contractions
2-3 mins apart
Consistent
Pressure

Dilation
10 cm

Effacement
100%
Station
+2 and beyond

Things to do

Changing Positions
Listening to body
Resting between
Breathing deep
Laboring down

On average a birther will push between 2-3 hours and change positions 6 times.

What are some tools that can help you with pushing?

____

____

____

____

Chapter 6
Baby Earthside

You

did

it!

BOOK OF LABOR

Chapter 7: Placenta

Complete and feeling pressure

Feelings

Accomplished
Chills/Shakes
Oxytocin surge

Contractions

3-8 minutes
Similar to Early Labor

Things to do

Skin to Skin
Breast/Chestfeed
Rest
Listening to body

What are your plans for your placenta?

____

____

____

____

Obstacles: VBAC

VBAC

Successful VBAC Rate	80%
Risk of Uterine Rupture	~0.75%
Risk of Hysterectomy	0.23%
Risk of Blood Loss	1.89%

Repeat Cesarean

Risk of Hysterectomy	1.4 %
Risk of Blood Transfusion	1.53 %
Risk of Placenta Accreta	0.31 %
"Major" Complications	4.3 %
Risk of Scarring	21.6 %

What is your VBAC Calcultor Percentage?

___%

Remember that there are many factors that go into this percentage

C-section Incision Types

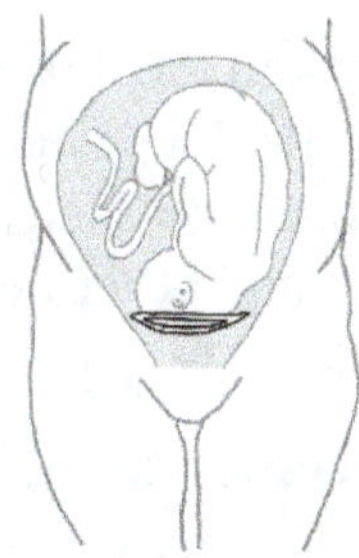 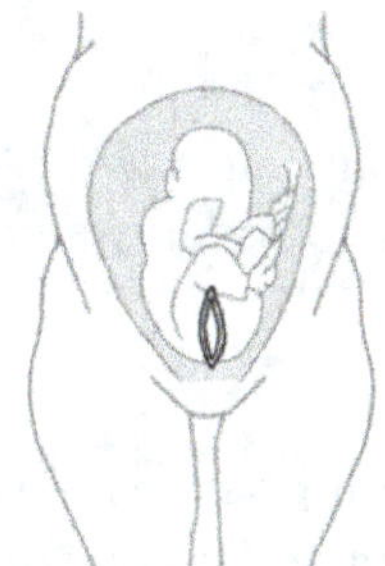 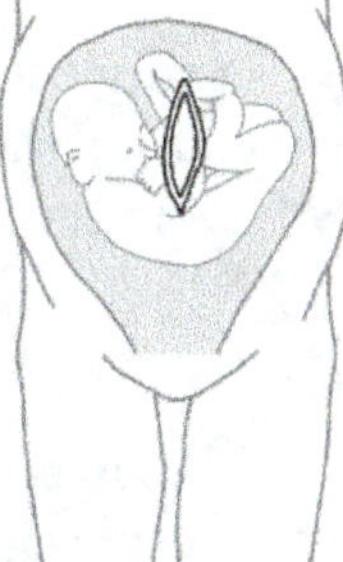 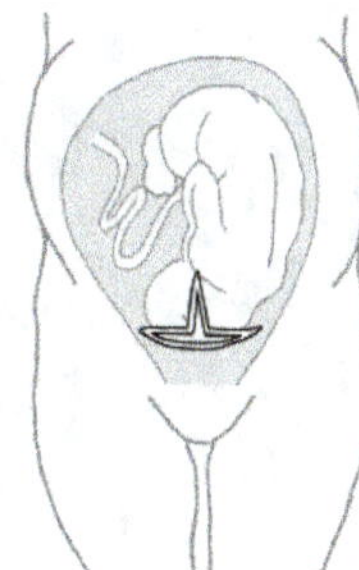 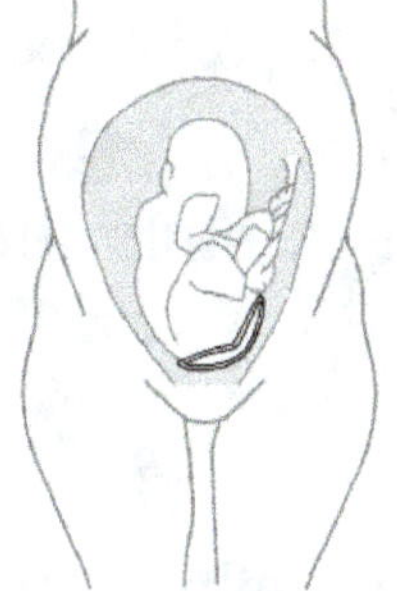

Low-Transverse
Most common incision type

Low-Vertical
Much like a classical incision but performed in the lower part of the uterine segment.

Classical
Most common type in the early 1900's. Still used sometimes when a rapid C-section is required or for premature, breech, or transverse babies.

Inverted T
Typically happens when a surgeon needs more room to get the baby out.

Inverted J
Can be used when a surgeon needs more room to get the baby out, sometimes happens by accident.

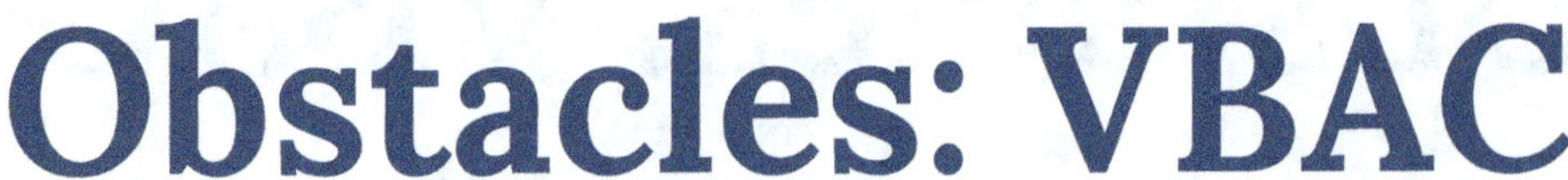

Obstacles: VBAC

Match the Intervention

BONUS: Circle the interventions that should never be used if you are going for a VBAC

Pitocin

Anesthetic placed in spine; reduces or sometimes eliminates the ability to move on your lower half. Can cause blood pressure issues; can stall labor-especially if given too soon.

AROM/Amniotomy

An amnihook is used to break the waters within the uterus. Studies show this does not reduce the time spent in labor.

Epidural

Synthetic version of oxytocin; disrupts the body's natural wave of hormones-BUT-can be responsibly when needed

Continuous Fetal Monitoring

Infused the uterus with sterile saline to increase the water around the baby improving the cushion baby is in the womb. Can improve cord compression scenarios.

Amnioinfusion

Care provider tells Birther to start pushing based on dilation vs waiting for the Birther to feel "Pushy". Can lead to long pushing and failure to descends.

Sweeping Membranes

A surgical cut to the perineum and the muscle beneath it during the pushing stage. Can be done necessarily but is often done to reduce pushing time. Can cause scarring and other nerve damage.

Directed Pushing

Lower your chances of needing a formal induction if your pregnancy goes on too long and you and your care provider decide that you want a formal induction. This can help prevent needing medications for an induction. 9% of mothers will have their water break at the same time.

Episiotomy

Your baby's heartbeat is checked all the time. Elastic belts hold two flat devices (called sensors) on your belly. One sensor records the baby's heart rate. The other shows how long your contractions last.

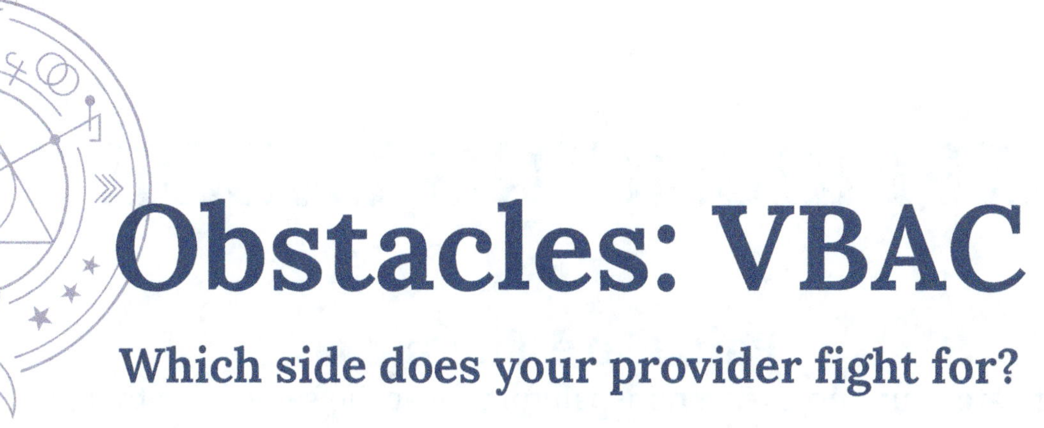

Obstacles: VBAC

Which side does your provider fight for?

VBAC Friendly

- [ ] No arbitrary restrictions on length of gestation
- [ ] Induction or augmentation are options if medically necessary or advisable
- [ ] No weight guesstimates used to discourage you from VBAC
- [ ] As long as Birther and baby are doing well, labor does not have time limits
- [ ] Encourages laboring outside of the hospital longer to avoid unnecessary interventions
- [ ] Low cesarean and high VBAC rates
- [ ] Supports VBAmC
- [ ] Can guarantee that they, or an equally supportive provider will be the one to attend your birth

VBAC Tolerant

- [ ] Must go into labor by Due date
- [ ] Won't induce or augment under any circumstance
- [ ] Baby must be under X lbs
- [ ] Must progress X cm/hr
- [ ] Must come to the hospital in early labor
- [ ] Epidural placed "just in case"
- [ ] Internal fetal monitoring and/or intrauterine pressure catheter required
- [ ] Must have double layer sutures
- [ ] Uses a VBAC calculator
- [ ] Shares a practice with other unsupportive providers that don't share their view and may not "let you"

EXPERIENCING LABOR

Pain Gate Theory

Activate your nerves in a non-painful way at the same time that you're experiencing pain, that that blocks the pain signals from reaching your brain.

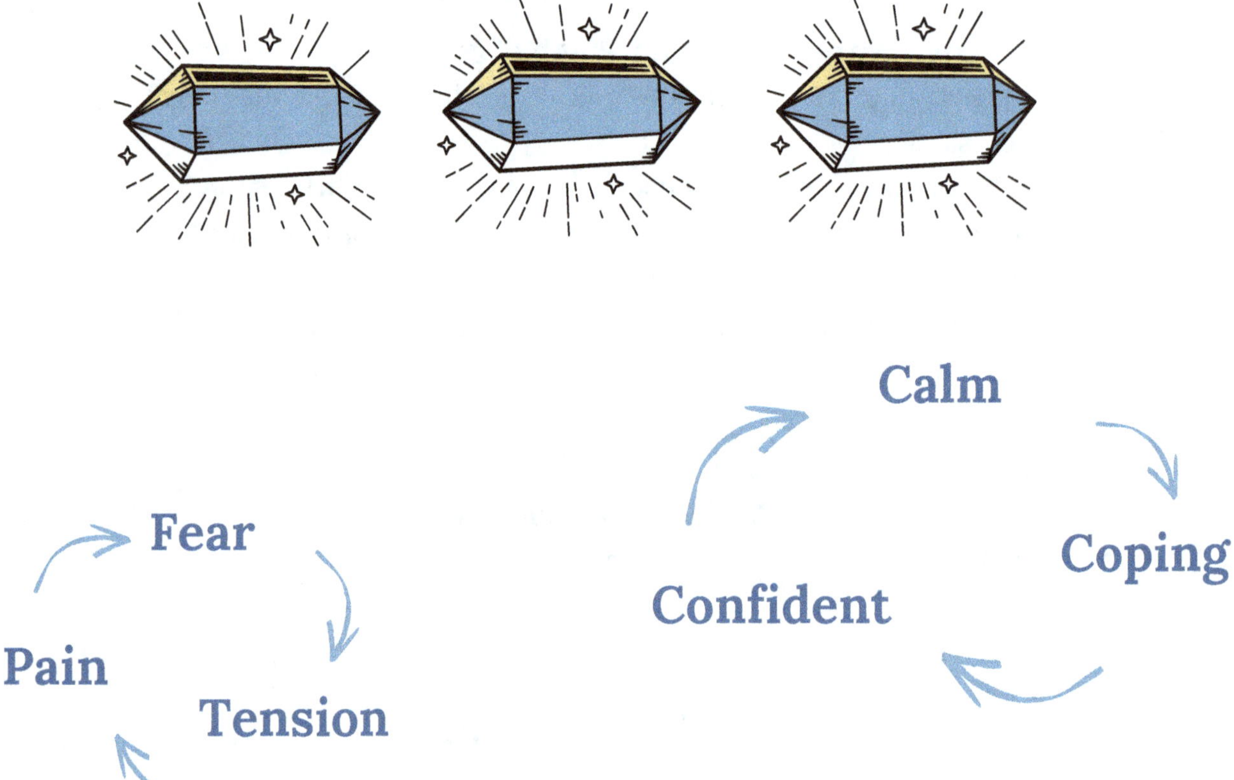

Pain Vortex

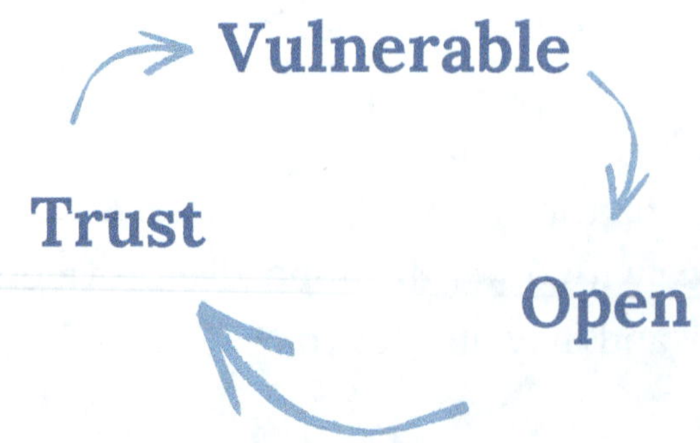

TOOLS FOR LABOR

Unmedicated
Circle your favorite

Comb

Birthing ball

Birth Stool

Walking

Dancing

Water

Jiggle

Aromatherapy

Breath

Growling

HypnoBirth/Babies

Acupuncture

Tens Unit

Double Hip Squeeze

Brushing Teeth

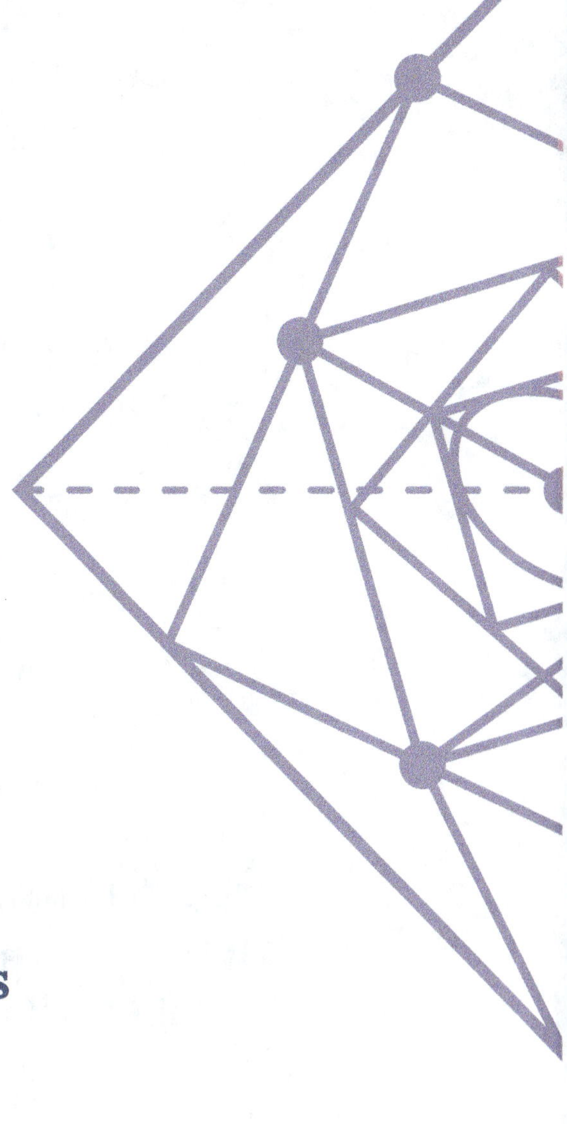

TOOLS FOR LABOR

Medicated

Epidural

an injection in your back to stop you
feeling pain in part of your body

Injected Opioids

used for acute, acute-on-chronic, or chronic
pain that cannot be controlled by other pain
management options

Nitrous Oxide

nitrous oxide is not a strong analgesic.
Birthers who use nitrous oxide during labor
may still have an awareness of labor pain.

Saline Shots

These injections are given into the person's lower back.
The onset of pain relief is fast, so it works pretty quickly
within about two minutes, and the pain management
effects can last as long as two hours

Therapeutic Rest

Therapeutic rest in labor involves administration of
parenteral analgesics in early or prodromal labor to
relieve the patient's discomfort

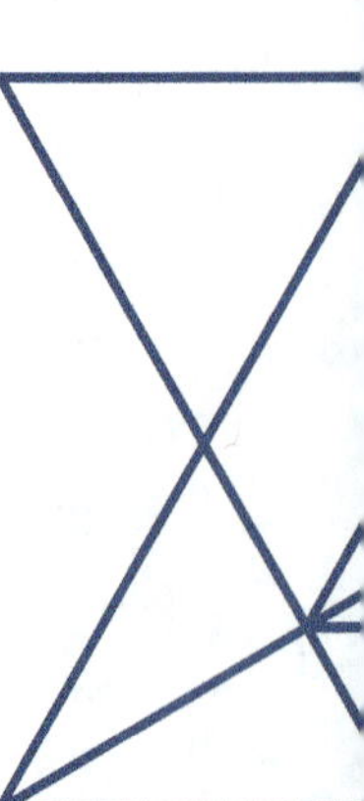

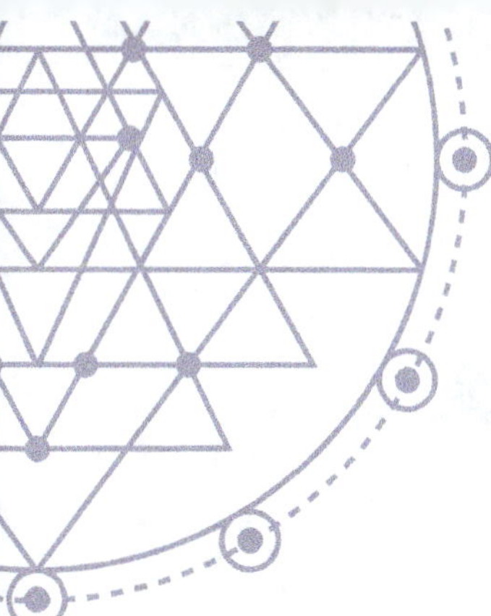

Mental Games

Catastrophe Game

____

____

____

____

Nothing Changes

____

____

____

____

Your own mental game
Please write the rules the game your mind loves to play

____

____

____

____

____

____

Birth Trauma

Stats say ___ birthing people will have a traumatic birth

Who is at risk?

__________ complications
Birthing Interventions
Babies needing ________ care
People with significant injuries
People with existing _______ problems
People with previous trauma and abuse People from marginalized backgrounds
NO ONE IS IMMUNE!!

___ of people try a treatment approach and it doesn't work

Write 4 resources you can use in case of emergency

Party Members

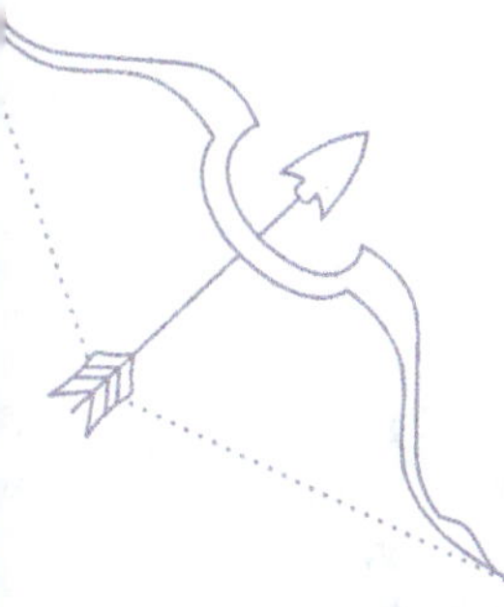

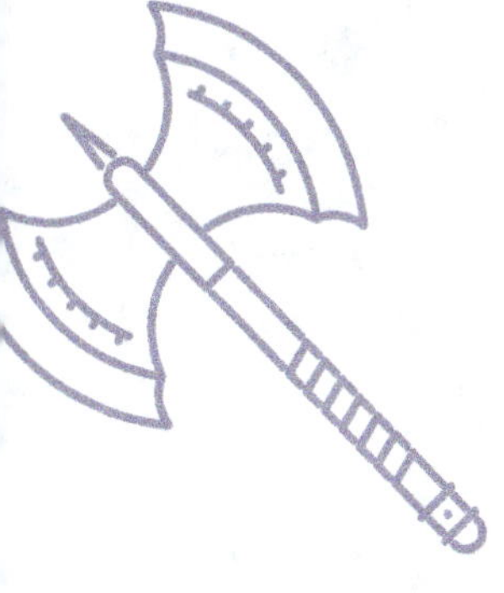

Name your qualities and skills only you
can bring to this quest

____

____

____

Name 3 birth wishes you hope to fulfill
during this quest

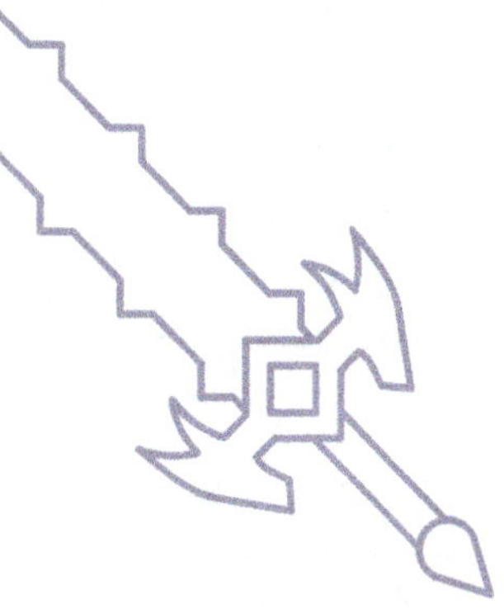

____

____

____

Advocating

B _______________

R _______________

A _______________

I _______________

N _______________

Boundary Riffing

Write down your favorites

____

____

____

____

Fear Release

Fear Bubbles

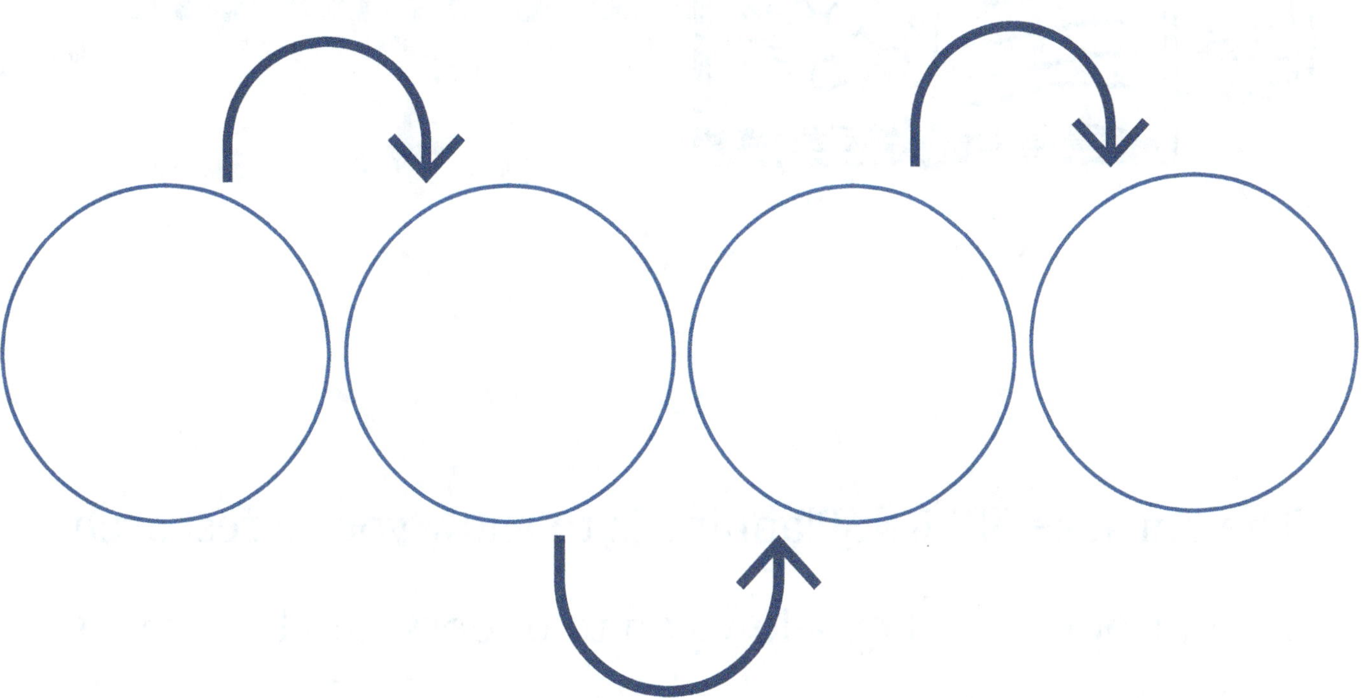

Breath Work

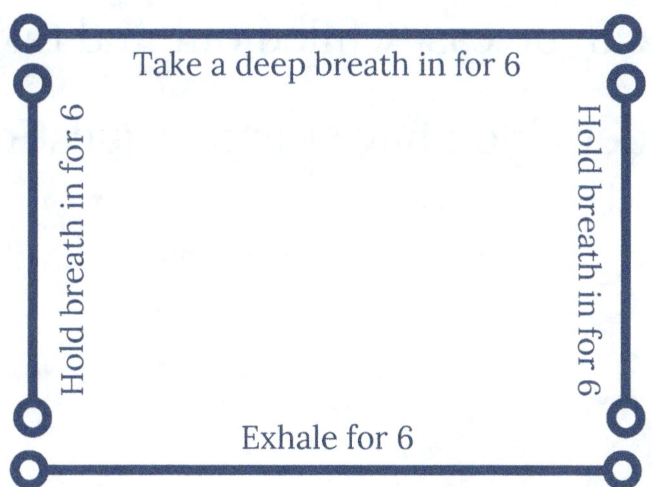

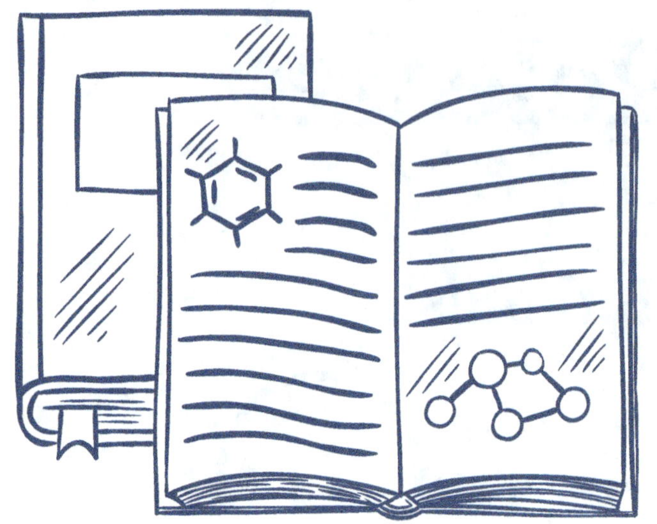

Birth Research

The purpose of Birth Planning is to allow you to research all your options. They allow you to understand backroads incase your journey hits a plot twist. Please take the time to use our light version of a birth plan for your own journey. It can be easily filled out and taken to your provider if you have further questions....

Birth Choices

Birth Name:

Partner:

Provider:

Pediatrician:

Baby Name:

Augmentation & Monitoring

- ☐ Movement
- ☐ Artificial rupture of membranes (AROM)
- ☐ Pitocin
- ☐ Cervidil/Cytotec
- ☐ Membrane Sweep
- ☐ a clear or lowered drape
- ☐ to have a slow delivery
- ☐ Intermittent Monitoring
- ☐ Continuous Monitoring
- ☐ Internal Monitoring

Pushing

- ☐ Perfer to wait to push until I feel the urge
- ☐ Mirror
- ☐ Coached Pushing
- ☐ Forceps
- ☐ Touch my baby's head as it crowns
- ☐ Pull baby out myself
- ☐ Have my partner catch baby
- ☐ Natural Tearing
- ☐ Use a variety of positions during pushing

Pain Management

- ☐ Movement
- ☐ Counter Pressue
- ☐ Water: Tub or Shower
- ☐ Nitrous Oxide
- ☐ Birth Ball
- ☐ Tens Unit
- ☐ Tramadol/Opioids
- ☐ Local Anesthesia
- ☐ Epidural

Baby & After Birth Care

- ☐ Delayed Cord Clamping
- ☐ Skin to Skin
- ☐ Vitamin K Shot/Drops
- ☐ Eye Ointment
- ☐ Breast/Chestfeeding ☐ Formula
- ☐ Pitocin for bleeding
- ☐ Donate Placenta/Cord Blood
- ☐ Keeping Placenta
- ☐ Keep Baby in Room

Birth Choices

Birth Name:

Partner:

Provider:

Pediatrician:

Baby Name:

Prior to Birth, I would like

- ☐ to meet with members of the OR team who will be with me during delivery
- ☐ an explanation of the procedure before I am taken to the OR
- ☐ an explanation of the medications that will be used
- ☐ my partner/spouse/family member/doula to accompany me in the delivery room

For Pain Relief, I would like

- ☐ Epidural
- ☐ Spinal
- ☐ General Anesthesia

During Birth, I would like

- ☐ to wear my own labor and delivery gown
- ☐ to choose the music playing in OR
- ☐ ECG leads placed on my back
- ☐ my support to take pictures/video
- ☐ the procedure explained as it happens
- ☐ a clear or lowered drape
- ☐ to have a slow delivery
- ☐ Side Conversation limited
- ☐ No Students

Immediately following Birth, I would like

- ☐ my partner in the OR to announce the gender of our baby
- ☐ to delay cord clamping
- ☐ my spouse/partner to cut the umbilical cord
- ☐ immediate skin-to-skin on me or my partner
- ☐ vaginal seeding to be performed
- ☐ to have measurements/assessments performed while the baby is on my chest if they are needed immediately
- ☐ do not give me sedatives after the birth
- ☐ to see and touch the placenta and cord
- ☐ to have the opportunity to breastfeed in the OR

During Recovery, I would like

- ☐ a lactation consultant to visit
- ☐ my other children to come in to meet the new baby
- ☐ family to visit within 1-3 hours after birth
- ☐ my IV, catheter, ECG leads, etc. removed as soon as possible
- ☐ to eat and get up to use the restroom as soon as I feel ready and able to following delivery
- ☐ Limited interaction with nursing staff in night hours to allow rest and bonding
- ☐ a breast pump accessible in my room

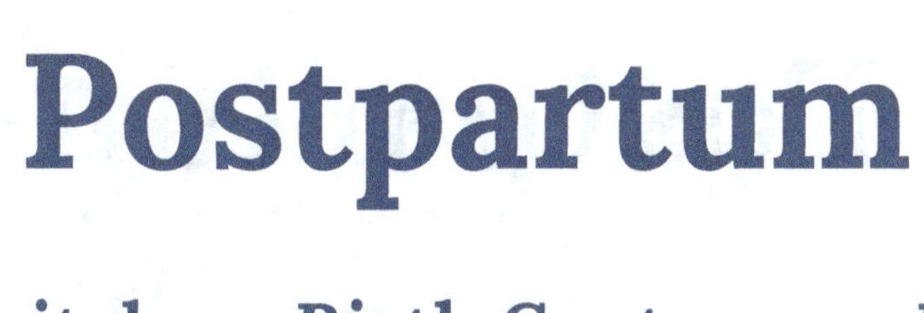

Postpartum

	Hospital	Birth Center	Home
60 Minutes	Pitocin if needed Fundus Massage Skin to Skin Baby Tests	Pitocin if needed Fundus Massage Skin to Skin Meal Provided	Pitocin if needed Fundus Massage Skin to Skin Meal Provided
60 Hours	Typically Home Bleeding continues Milk shifting Hormone shifts/baby blues	Visit from Provider Bleeding continues Milk shifting Hormone shifts/baby blues	Visit from Provider Bleeding continues Milk shifting Hormone shifts/baby blues
60 Days	6 week postpartum appt 45-60 days ovulation occurs Cleared for usual activities	6 week postpartum appt 45-60 days ovulation occurs Cleared for usual activities	6 week postpartum appt 45-60 days ovulation occurs Cleared for usual activities

What are some of your plans for postpartum?

____

____

____

____

____

Postpartum

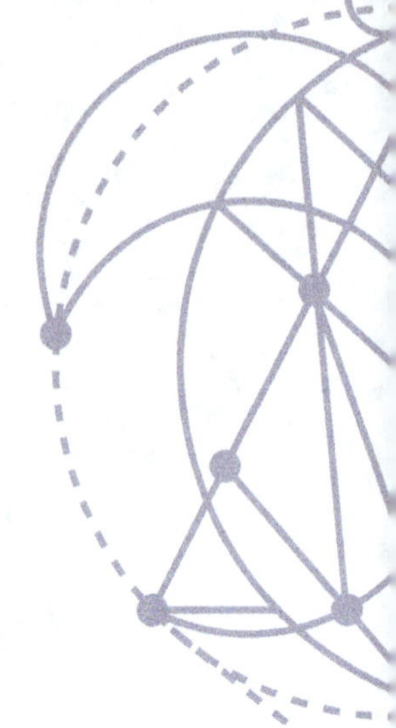

**S
N
O
W
B
A
L
L**

Resources that you'll need

____

____

____

____

Presenting of your Certificate of Birth Wisdom

Notes

Notes

Notes

Notes

Notes

Notes

Notes

Notes

Notes

Notes

Notes